7-Day

Weight Loss Challenge

7-Day

WEIGHT LOSS

CHALLENGE

Lose Weight In 7 Days

CHALLENGE SELF

http://www.ChallengeSelf.com

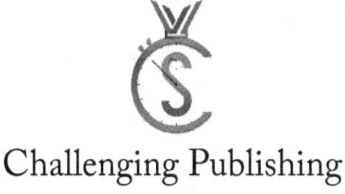

Challenging Publishing

ISBN 978-1-523-39948-2

Printed in the United States of America

First Edition

YOUR OVERVIEW:

<u>Your Instructions:</u>

How to Best Approach This

This book is not meant to be read entirely in one sitting, but for over the span of each day.

Why? The reasons are relatively simple. We do want you to benefit from the information, which will take time to process, and we do not want to overwhelm you with all the applications of what you will learn. At the same time, we don't want to make this another breezy one-time read, and then you're off to do something else, forgetting your new knowledge without ever applying it to anything.

Now you probably will be eager and tempted to go through this all in one sitting, but we're encouraging you to take it slow. Remember that the best way to approach this is <u>one day</u> at a time. Do not move on to the next day until you have completed its previous day(s).

This approach is effective because if you truly want to improve, you need to remain grounded in the process. There is no such thing as a magic pill; there is continuous conditioned improvement. Rome wasn't built in a day. Likewise, none of the top performers, best athletes, and successful people in the world have gotten to where they are in a day. Breaking things up into separate days supports an ongoing process and builds upon each previous day's progress to bring it all home in the end.

Of course, each individual's experience will be different. You may or may not accomplish your goal after the entire trial is over. In that case, you can repeat it all again starting from Day 1 to the last day.

If you commit yourself, you will see improvement. Are you ready to proceed on to your challenges? Then let's begin!

P.S. If you ever need to contact us, you can always reach out to us at our official website:

http://www.ChallengeSelf.com

<u>Your Challenge:</u>

Lose Weight

Millions of people (men and women) around the world are obsessed with losing weight. But what are the facts behind this craze? How do we know if our weight is actually healthy or not?

If you've ever wondered this, here's your <u>answer</u>: scientific research backs the fact that we need to be a certain weight in order to be considered healthy.

Obviously there isn't a universal weight that applies to everyone, so to calculate for yourself, you have to understand your **Body Mass Index (or BMI)**. Your BMI helps you estimate your *total body fat*, and is considered a good indicator of your weight-related risks.

Here's an example to give you a clearer idea of how this index works: When your BMI is between 18.5 and 24.9, your weight is considered **normal**. If your BMI is 25, you're considered **overweight**, and by 30 or over, you're considered **obese**.

In the US alone (according to the National Health and Nutrition Examination Survey), more than 2 out of 3 adults are considered overweight, and 1/3 (34.9% of the population) are considered obese. These numbers are alarming, and they designate just how badly we eat in this country.

And, as if these facts weren't bewildering enough, the dieter-to-be also has to deal with all the scientific researchers urging us to lose weight—eat better, exercise more, etc.—and all the companies that spring out of nowhere, claiming to have the next big thing **YOU** need to use for weight loss: it's revolutionary, it's an ancient civilization secret, it's a product you can use to "never have to exercise again!"

But you can't deny the fact that both the businessmen and the scientists are right: when you're slim, you're more confident, more comfortable, and overall more attractive to others. They know what we all want—to look good and feel healthy.

To achieve this, then, it's all about how you envision your own weight-loss journey. Losing weight is an objective— one that you have to organize in order to get satisfactory results. But it's not just a scientific exercise—it should be personal because it involves your body and requires changes in *your* habits and *your* life.

This is all your deal. You have to believe in yourself, push and motivate yourself, and keep yourself from giving up when things look tough. People aren't necessarily going to encourage you like you want them to, so it's important that *you* believe in your decision to lose weight—no matter what.

And be honest, wouldn't you rather be healthy and look good than feel guilty every time you sit down to eat? To diet successfully, you first need the confidence boost that comes with losing weight and keeping it off, and secondly, you need to understand that your eating habits and your weight are actually health risks. By eating healthily, you can improve your quality of life and reduce your risks of diseases and other health complications.

So, make sure you keep in mind that the number one method for weight-loss success is to make it your own personal battle. This is for you—don't do it to try to impress others.

To see how serious you are about losing weight, try taking the following quiz. And be honest with you answers; you don't have to share this with anyone. Ever.

Pick the most appropriate answer:

1.) How long did your last weight-loss program last?

a.) A week.

b.) A month.

c.) I'm still at it after 2 years.

2.) Did you work hard to eat healthier last time you decided to lose weight?

a.) No. I can eat what I want as long as I exercise, right?

b.) Yes, but after a month I couldn't resist the cravings anymore.

c.) Yes, and I feel it's the best decision I've ever made.

3.) What pushed you to want to lose weight?

a.) I'm tired of looking frumpy, and my hot friend told me about a new diet that really worked for her.

b.) Just to see if I was up to the task.

c.) I realized my lifestyle wasn't healthy.

4.) How many times do you work out per week?

a.) I don't remember—it's been a while.

b.) Whenever I feel like it.

c.) Exactly four times a week.

5.) How many meals do you have on a normal day?

a.) I've lost count—do I have to include burgers and snacks?

b.) Maybe 5. It depends on the day.

c.) Exactly 3 a day—I try to respect timing for all my meals.

*If you've picked mostly **A**, you're just a follower when it comes to weight loss. It's never been a personal ambition for you, and unless someone close to you decides to start a new diet, you're content to keep things the way they are. You should start looking at where your life is heading and how your choices are impacting your body. Ask yourself if you're happy with your diet (the way you eat) and if there's any way you can switch this around. If you've never understood how other people can diet so successfully, read on and find out now!

If you've picked mostly **B, you have a problem when it comes to planning a weight-loss routine. You have to understand that weight-loss is something very difficult—something demands a lot of change and determination. If you don't follow a plan or a well elaborated weekly/daily program, it's just not worth starting any diet right now. Perhaps you should take a minute to read through this 7-day program and learn more about how it should be done.

***If you've picked mostly **C,** you're a weight-loss guru my friend! You're a determined person; your character is that of a "go-getter". Your secret is that you have faith in you and in your decisions, and most of all, you're able to recognize and work on your weight problem. It might be weight gained during pregnancy or weight gained due to too much partying during the holidays—whatever it is, you just don't give up. You get things done, and right away. But there might still be a few tricks and tips you can learn, so read on and enjoy this 7-day program.

DAY 1:

Begin the Mental Prep

Define Your Goals

One of the reasons people often fail or give up on dieting is that they never took the time to sit down and actually prepare a realistic, step-by-step weight-loss program. Make no mistake: this *is* an important step.

By writing up a strategy, you're actualizing your objectives and goals and making sure your plan will work for you. Everyone has their own individual needs, so you can't just imitate your "hot friend's" diet or one you saw on TV. That specific diet may have worked for her/him, but you have to do what works for *you*.

So, let's get to the basics of building your weight-loss goal and creating the plan you'll use to achieve it.

Step 1: Determine Your Ideal Weight

As discussed earlier, you'll need to start by calculating your BMI to give you an idea of how much you should normally weigh. Okay, so how do you do that? Well, you basically have to multiply your weight and divide it by your height (multiplied by itself first).

Don't worry, it's a simple mathematical equation. It'll end up looking like this:

BMI = *(Weight in lbs. x 703) / (Height in inches)* x *(Height in inches)*

The number you come up with lets you know where you stand and how much you need to lose (remember, indexes between 18.5 and 24.9 designate a normal weight, and 25 or over is considered overweight).

Step 2: Set Milestone Deadlines for Yourself

When you're done calculating your BMI, you have to determine **how much time you'll need to lose that weight**. Be realistic here—people that set themselves extreme goals tend to fail, so make sure you give yourself a realistic time period for a reasonable amount of weight. Not sure what sort of time limit you should give yourself?

Here's a tip: You normally start seeing your weight drop within 2 weeks of starting a new diet. If you're *just* working out, you'll start seeing results (like a more defined silhouette and probably some weight loss) after about 2 to 3 months. So, when you set your goals, keep in mind that: It. Will. Take. Time. In other words, you're going to have to be patient and also take your time.

So, you'll definitely need to plan for a medium-to-long-term goal here. In this case, your best strategy would be to set your goals by the month, for up to 6 month periods.

For instance, if you want to lose **20 pounds**, you could aim to lose **10 pounds** in the *first 3 months,* then the **remaining 10** by the *6th month.* As you can probably see, the deal is to cut your main goal into smaller chunks that are more manageable and easier to visualize.

Step 3: Gather Your Tools

What are your weight-loss tools? By "tools" we mean the activities and life-changing decisions you'll have to make in order to lose weight.

Right now, though, we're specifically talking about your choice of workout (yoga, cardio, aerobics, etc.), your choice of diet, the number of times you actually eat per day (3, 4, 8 times?), and the motivation you'll need to keep going. Again, be realistic here and don't try to fool yourself.

Determine your exercise program for the first 3 months based on how often you *honestly* think you can work out every week (can you do it 5 times a week? 3 times?). To make sure you see results in at least 3 months, however, make sure you work out at least 3 times a week and at most 5.

According to Shawn Arent, an exercise scientist at Rutgers University, one should exercise a minimum of *three days* per week—which implies that anything below that number just isn't enough. It's something to remember when you set up your weight-loss program.

Step 4: Maintain Your Weight

How do you keep the weight off? From the very beginning of your program, you're going to have to be prepared to make these changes a permanent part of your lifestyle. No more breakfast at Taco Bell, no more microwavable dishes, and no more sodas. *Ah boohoo, but fret not!* Get ready to substitute those habits with healthier alternative choices such as water, home-cooked meals, regular workouts, etc.

You should understand now why preparation and planning are stressed as so important for a successful outcome. Only a well-thought-out plan (don't put your expectations too high) and a reachable goal (medium to long-term) can help you build the endurance and determination you'll need to not only succeed your weight-loss goals but maintain them.

Setting up goals, especially when it comes to something as life-changing as losing weight and healthier living, is like drafting out plans for a building. An architect takes the time to make sure his plans and blueprints are logical and workable, while a designer starts off "from his imagination." When the time comes and the buildings are finished, the architect's well-planned building stands firm, while the designer's building experiences all sorts of health problems and reliability issues.

Exercise: Plan Your Roadmap

So, to make sure your weigh-loss roadmap is on track out and won't wobble the minute it's put to use, take a few minutes now and draft one up.

1.) First, calculate your **BMI.**

Example: If you're 180 pounds and 5'4," your BMI would be:

(Weight in lbs. x 703) / (Height in inches) x (Height in inches) = (180 x 703) / (64 x 64) = 126540 / 4096 = 30.89.

Since your end result is slightly over 30, you can tell that you're definitely over the limit for a healthy weight.

2.) After calculating your BMI, determine how much weight you want to lose overall, then break it down into

achievable milestones. If, for instance, you wanted to lose <u>15 pounds</u>, you could aim to lose **3 pounds a month** for 5 months.

3.) Determine <u>how long it should take you to see results</u>. In other words, how long do you want to be on your program? *Six months, a year?* It all depends on you. You can make it as hard or as (relatively) easy as you think you need to.

4.) Next, determine the tools you'll use to help you. To set up a 5-times-a-week exercise program, for instance, you could organize it on these lines:

Monday: Aerobics

Tuesday: Yoga session

Wednesday: Weight-lifting

Thursday: Pilates

Friday: 20-minute run

(*This week we'll be walking you through an optimum workout routine, but for planning purposes, just remember to keep your exercise sessions to a minimum of 3 times a week and a maximum of 5 times. Too much exercise and you'll burn yourself out before the first week is up; not enough exercise and you won't be burning enough calories. One way to organize your workouts is to schedule your exercise times during the 5 work days, leaving yourself the weekend to rest. It's important to keep rest a part of your program, too.)

5.) Lastly, you'll need to build strategies tailored to you personally to keep that weight off once you've actually started losing it.

- For example, you can set your bedtime earlier so you're not tempted by late-night snacking, or you can decide to replace your soda with water from now on. Examine your lifestyle and habits and determine which ones are keeping you from realizing your goals. Those are the ones that need to go.

7-Day Weight Loss Challenge

DAY 2:

Regenerate Your Metabolic Powers

Start the Fight from Within

Day 1 was all about being mentally and strategically prepared. Now that you've got your plan down, it's time to move from *mental* to *physical* preparation. And the first thing you've got to work on to help your body make the most of this program is your metabolism.

So, how does your metabolism affect weight loss? It's simple. A healthy person (one who's active and doesn't eat processed foods all the time) burns calories at a natural rate—and the faster your metabolism, the faster your body burns those calories.

But the metabolism tends to start slowing down once a person reaches a certain age, generally around 25 (especially in women). That's why teenagers (most of them) have a slim figure—their bodies, when accustomed to a certain non-toxic rhythm, burn calories at a steady rate every day. Specialists, such as Obi Obadicke, a celebrity trainer and fitness expert, say that from age 25, the metabolism of an average person starts slowing down at a rate of 2 to 4% every year.

But if you're past that age, don't despair. There are many ways to increase your metabolism, one of which we'll discuss here: **the hot water treatment.**

Don't worry, it's not as intimidating as it sounds. Scientists have discovered that, by drinking hot water in the morning and before your meals, you can increase your body temperature, helping you detox faster and boosting your metabolism at the same time. And, as it turns out, this technique is even more effective when combined with a good workout schedule.

Chinese people are known to drink hot beverages with all their meals (there are various amazing reasons, all supported by science) to control appetite, at the same time protecting organ functions and increasing energy levels is one reason why in Asian cultures obesity is less common.

Scientists like Dr. Michael Wald, director of Nutritional Services at Integrated Medicine and Nutrition in Mount Kisco, New York, attest that hot water can in fact increase body temperature and slightly increase the metabolic rate, causing your body to burn more calories throughout the day. Sounds perfect for weight loss, right?

Exercise: The Hot Cleanse

So, to make use of this new knowledge, make hot water part of your weight-loss program and add it to your schedule following the plan below:

–Drink 1 cup of hot water (if plain water doesn't appeal to you, you can add a slice of lime or lemon) as soon as you wake up in the morning.

–Drink 1 glass of hot water before each meal (lunch and dinner).

–To finish off the cleanse, add 1 more glass of water around 4 pm, and another before you go to bed. In all, it amounts to 5 glasses of hot water a day (added to the cool or room temperature water we assume you normally drink).

From Day 2 onward, then, your assignment will be to continue drinking hot water (lime or lemon flavored, if you prefer) throughout the day. Make sure you take your first cup in the morning before anything else, then one *before* or *with* every meal, substituting what you would normally have.

- How do you feel after your first glass of hot water?

- Do you feel lighter or more active during the day?

- Does your food seem to be digested faster? Explain.

*It's important that you make this schedule part of your daily routine. The "hot water treatment" will not only help you digest and boost your metabolism but it will also make your workout routine that much more effective. And let's face it, how much easier could losing weight get? So, make sure you drink that hot water all the way up to Day 7.

DAY 3:

Reprogram Your Food Channel

Changing the Eating Habit

Day 3 is when you start dealing with the most difficult part of the weight-loss program: **food**. It's possible, though, that this difficulty is mostly mental, because people tend to associate dieting or weight loss with depriving oneself of tasty food—which certainly doesn't have to be the case.

The type of food to eat: The first requirement of a good diet plan is that it be healthy, there. (No-brainer.) So it should be made up of foods you can enjoy, with a lot of fruit and vegetables, lean meat, seafood, beans, nuts, and small amounts of healthy grains.

Although the plan is to make your meals as enjoyable as possible, you do need to make sure that processed foods make up a very small percentage of your diet (since they're high in sugar and carbs and have little or no nutrients at all).

Keep in mind with a diet it's best to take baby steps. If you resolve not to buy any more cakes or cookies, for instance, it doesn't mean you can't have a slice of birthday cake when you go to a party. It's all about setting reasonable limits. If you try to go cold turkey and deny yourself even a crumb of cake, you're more likely to break your diet completely and give up altogether. So, an occasional treat, especially if it's something you can't bring home to tempt you, might actually be more of a help than a hindrance here.

Getting the Nutrition

Remember, *baby steps*. The best way to achieve a better diet is to slowly switch your normal (aka unhealthy or evil) foods for healthier alternatives.

Again, planning can help you here. Before you start your new eating program, draw yourself up a table, listing the nutrients you need every day from your food. It might sound involved, but don't worry: we've listed some ideas to get you started.

- Start with carbohydrates (you won't need many of these), protein (for building and repairing tissue), healthy fats (for providing energy), vitamins and minerals (to maintain optimal health), and water (which enables vital bodily functions). Once you have your categories listed on your table, list healthy foods you can eat for each category. For an example, take a look at Table A below:

Table A: Example healthy food substitutes chart.

CARBOHYDRATES	Dried fruit, sweet potatoes, unprocessed grains, vegetables, legumes, beans, fruits, nuts, and yogurt.
PROTEIN	Fish, Lean chicken, Cheese, lean beef and veal, yogurt, milk, pork loin, tofu, eggs (especially egg whites), nuts and seeds (pumpkin, squash, and watermelon seeds).
FATS	Beef, beef fat, veal, lamb, pork, lard, poultry fat, butter, cream, milk, cheeses and other dairy products made from whole and 2 percent milk.
VITAMINS AND MINERALS	Meats, fish, and poultry. However, you can get zinc and iron in dried beans, seeds, nuts, and leafy green vegetables like kale.
WATER	In general, all food has some water in it; with fruit and vegetables containing 80 to 98 percent water. Eating vegetables such as cucumbers, tomatoes, jicama, beets, carrots or celery with a meal or snack is one of the easiest ways to improve your hydration. Other than that, don't forget to drink the recommended 8 glasses of water a day.

Substituting the Old for the New

When you've completed your table, start another list—this time made up of typical foods you eat when not on a diet.

Example: fried chicken, red meat, French fries, pizza, ice cream, soda . . . and all those other tasty foods filled with salt, sugar, and other additives (such as microwavable meals).

Once you've finished this list, start substituting these meals with ones from the previous "healthy" list.

For instance, if you're used to snacking on a Snickers bar and a big bag of chips, substitute them with a home-made fruit salad, nuts, yogurt, or a banana; instead of two pieces of fried chicken, you could make it two small pieces of lean chicken (chicken breasts), and so on. As long as you keep your substitute portions a reasonable size and stick to your healthy foods chart, you're good to go. For more examples, see the table below:

Table B: A list of typical unhealthy meals taken during the week vs. their more healthy substitutes.

MEALS	MEALS NORMALLY EATEN	HEALTHY SUBSTITUTES
BREAKFAST	Pancakes, French pastries, coffee.	Fruit salad, eggs, 1 orange, 1 cup of green tea.
LUNCH	Meal at McDonald, Double cheese sandwich with ham and eggs, cheesecake, soda.	A green salad, fish filet with steamed vegetables, water.
SNACKS (FROM 11 AM TILL 11 PM)	A bar of snickers, candy, caramel sundae, flavored chips, caramel popcorn, soda.	1 banana, a low fat yogurt, or some nuts. A glass of fruit juice.
DINNER	A whole pizza, lasagna, baked ham, mac and cheese. A milkshake for drink.	Beef stew (home made), grapes for desert and a glass of water.

The meals listed here are typical examples of unhealthy meals and their healthier alternatives. But remember, these are just examples. When you draw your own table, feel free to write in your own alternatives—as long as they come from your healthy foods list, of course.

Now that you've worked out the basics of what you can and can't eat, it's time to move on to the next stage of diet planning:

Timing is Everything

Frequency of meals during the day: In the last section you looked at the *what* of dieting, so now it's time to look at the *when* and *how much*.

You might never have thought of *when* you eat as being that important, but, according to studies, a person stops digesting food properly after 9 o'clock at night—in other words, everything you put in after that is just fat waiting to get stored in the wrong place (*think about it*). It's also possible that this habit of overloading the stomach "after hours" could be the culprit for those people who experience stomach pains and constant constipation.

And, as if that in itself weren't enough, findings from an early 2015 study—published in the Journal of Obesity—also strongly suggest that *when* you take in your calories makes a difference in how you lose weight. A study of 93 overweight women, following a 1,400-calorie diet, led to the conclusion that those who ate a large breakfast (700 calories) and a light dinner (200 calories) lost more than twice as much weight as women who ate a 200-calorie breakfast and 700-calorie dinner.

To make it clearer (without counting the calories), dieters who ate more in the morning and less in the evening felt less hungry during the day and had lower blood levels of a hormone called ghrelin. Ghrelin is a hunger hormone that stimulates appetite, increases food intake, and promotes fat storage. (It turns out that this hormone increases after dieting, which may explain, in part, why it can be difficult to *keep* your weight down afterward.) Overall, the researchers discovered that eating a large meal late in the day disrupts the body's internal clock and promotes weight gain.

Also, in her book Woman Heal Thyself, Jeanne Elisabeth Blum, an acupressure specialist (a healing art that works by putting pressure on key healing points), states that the pericardium (a membrane enclosing the heart), is at its peak from 7 pm to 9 pm—around the time that the stomach is busy digesting. The pericardium helps the heart pump blood to the stomach for digestion, so at this point, you're still digesting your last meal—and you really don't need to throw another big one right on top of that.

So, pick a time before 9 pm—let's say 7 or 7:30 pm—during which you'll have your last meal. This will give your body plenty of time to digest the food and process the nutrients it needs to help you wake up "bloat-free" the next morning.

Set Your Eating Time

Now, within the timing we've established, you'll have to decide how many meals you're going to have in all. This decision will have to be a decisive one, though, because even after you've lost the targeted pounds, you'll have to keep to this eating frequency in order to sustain a healthy weight.

To set your schedule, first look at your current eating frequency (the number of times you eat per day when not on a diet). If it's more than 3 times, what you need to do—you'll probably hate it, but it's necessary—is go back to the basic 3 meals a day, with a small 4th meal added around the end of the afternoon.

This particular pattern is set up to establish a certain equilibrium in your eating and to train your body to sustain itself on only a few meals a day. To do this properly, and to allow your body to digest thoroughly between meals, you have to make sure you set equal gaps between your eating hours.

In other words, if you happen to have breakfast at 8:00 or 8:30 am, you need to make sure the rest of your meals are set at equal distances from each other so that your stomach has ample time to digest breakfast and be empty and ready for the next meal (you should also be feeling hungry again by this time).

So, here's how you're schedule may look:

–Eat breakfast between 8:00 and 8:30. Make it a healthy, well-balanced meal (such as one from **Table B** above). Also, remember that for optimum digestion, your breakfast should be bigger than your last meal of the day.

–Eat lunch at the traditional time (12-12:30 pm, exactly 4 hours after breakfast) when your stomach has digested breakfast thoroughly and you're hungry again.

–4 hours later (around 4-4:30 pm), sneak in your 4th meal or snack. This should consist of fresh veggies and dip (like baby carrots, broccoli, etc.), nuts, a tuna sandwich, yogurt, or any other snack item listed on the tables above.

–Finally, around 7-7:30 (keeping to the 9 pm "deadline"), have dinner.

Some people might not get why 4 meals are recommended here rather than the conventional 3. And it's a legitimate question, since, normally, people don't eat more than that every day. But with the gaps in time between those 3 meals, it's way too easy to develop cravings—and anyone who's ever dieted before knows how disastrous *that* can be. Therefore, eating 3 times a day can lower your blood sugar levels, leading you to eat even more than you would if you just slipped in a small 4th meal every day (often it leads you to crave sugar and processed foods). And there's just no way you can train yourself to eat properly under those circumstances.

The well-known fitness expert Jillian Michaels, known by many through the reality show "The Biggest Loser," advises her followers (on social media) to eat every 4 hours. She states that it maintains your energy levels, stabilizes your sugar, and guarantees better health. She also advises 4 meals: breakfast, lunch, a snack, and dinner. And let's face it, the way this woman looks should be testimonial enough for anyone!

Thus, get this diet in gear by eating balanced meals every 3 to 4 hours. You'll boost your metabolism and start noticing weight loss in no time!

Exercise: Create New Eating Routine

Keeping in mind the 4-meals-a-day frequency, use today to start substituting those meals with healthier alternatives. Here's a sample of what your daily menu can look like:

–Drink your glass of hot water when you get up in the morning, then (should be around 8:00 or 8:30), instead of having breakfast at McDonald's, have a bowl of oatmeal, garnished with plenty of chopped fruit, and a cup of tea.

–Around 12 pm (lunch), have your second glass of hot water, then a small salad as an entrée, followed by your main dish—some lean chicken and green beans—with fruit for desert.

−As a 4 o'clock snack, have a handful each of nuts and raisins (after you've had your third glass of hot water for the day).

−Around 7 pm, have your fourth glass of hot water and your main meal: a small portion of brown rice, pork chops fried in butter, and a helping of peas. (Remember, you want to keep your last meal smaller than your breakfast.)

After you've tried your healthier substitutes throughout the day, answer the following questions:

- How did you feel after eating this way all day? Explain.

- Where you able to keep to the 4-hour rule? Explain.

- Do you feel hungry during the 4 hours that separate your meals? Explain.

It's never easy to change your eating habits, but if you stick firmly to this plan, you'll find that it gets easier and easier over time. The 4-hour stretch between meals is something you should learn to accept as part of your normal routine, since it focuses on teaching you to eat *only* when you're hungry, thereby cutting out the superfluous calories which are ultimately converted to fat.

*As with the hot water routine, your new meal substitution exercise should become a daily habit. So, whenever meals are mentioned from now on, just remember that we're talking about your new healthy alternatives.

DAY 4:

Time to Sculpt Your Perfect Body

Get Physical

No matter how well you've been doing so far, boosting your metabolism and eating a healthy diet just isn't enough. To make your weight-loss program successful, you have to combine these things with a solid **exercise program**.

There are a dozen different ways to exercise: from running to swimming, playing tennis, simply registering to the gym, or (another simple option) doing it at home with personal workout videos. The selection is huge, so there's nothing limited about this part of the program. And, technically, just about any physical activity relating to a sport is good as long as it doesn't require you to overexert yourself too often.

But remember, with exercise—as with food—to be able to successfully keep it up, you have to be able enjoy it; your body shouldn't have to hurt too much and your heart shouldn't have to bear a whole lot of stress.

One way to get the full benefits of working out is to get your exercise in as early in the day as possible to really get energized for throughout the day. Think about it: you haven't worn yourself down yet, you're at your most motivated in the morning, and the adrenaline you secrete while working out helps improve your mood and fuel the rest of your day.

There is research that supports the benefits of working out first thing in the morning—especially for those of you who have a problem with consistency. According to Cedric

Bryant, PhD, chief science officer with the American Council on Exercise in San Diego, people who exercise in the morning adopt the routine easily and do very well when it comes to weight loss. What is there to lose?

And it's understandable that people have many obligations and don't necessarily have enough time in the morning, but it's important that you do your best to either *make* time or schedule your exercise days to avoid this problem. Few people have time to run to the gym in the afternoon, so the only time left to them is after work. The problem with this, though, is that getting that shot of adrenaline and increasing your heart rate that late in the evening can make going to sleep earlier *(remember that?)* a lot harder. It's something to think about when setting up your exercise plan.

Types of Workout

To help you with that plan, here's a list of dynamic workouts to consider for your new exercise routine:

–**Aerobics**: The American Heart Association and the American College of Sports Medicine recently published guidelines in which they recommend either 30 minutes of moderately intense aerobic exercise 5 days a week or 20 minutes of high-intensity aerobic exercise 3 days a week to maintain good health and reduce your risk of chronic disease.

–**Weight exercises**: According to Lisa Wheeler (fitness program director for DailyBurn), working out with weights helps you build strong bones, slows bone loss, increases strength and metabolism, improves glucose processing and lowers cholesterol, betters brain function, and can help you improve your overall health and wellness.

–**Yoga**: Developed in India, about 5,000 years ago, yoga not only helps you burn calories and tone muscles but it's also a total mind-body workout that combines strengthening and stretching poses with deep breathing, meditation, and relaxation. It has become popular in the US, not only as an exercise but also because it helps you feel better about yourself by improving blood circulation in your body.

–**Toning exercises**: A muscle toning exercise is a term that applies to any type of exercise that forces a muscle to travel its full range of motion while under resistance. An example of this type of exercise is a standing straight-bar biceps curl, which causes you to execute both concentric contractions (when a movement forces the muscle to shorten in length) and eccentric contractions (when the muscle is extended).

Each of these exercises has the advantage of making you sweat and work every bit of your body. They're all beneficial—and practically any exercise is going to work for you at the beginning of your program—so pick two or three of them to practice this week (one category at a time).

Remember, as well as working on your extra weight, exercising can also boost your self-confidence and enhance your mood. In fact, a study conducted in 2010 at the University of California, San Francisco, made the discovery that exercising might actually work on a cellular level to reverse the toll of stress on our aging process. The researchers found that stressed-out women who exercised vigorously for an average of 45 minutes over a 3-day period had cells that showed fewer signs of aging as compared to women who were stressed but inactive.

Exercise: Create New Workout Routine

To kick that extra weight *and* the stress in your life, add the following routine to your daily program:

–Starting between 5:30 and 6:30 am, work out for at least 30 minutes (but no more than 60). You'll get an exercise plan later on, but today try starting with aerobics.

–Drink some cool water immediately after exercising, then have your first glass of hot water, eat breakfast, and get prepared for the day.

Follow the same pattern each time you work out, and, by the end of week one, you should start noticing some changes in your mood, weight, and body.

- How do you feel after this first day of exercising? Explain.

- At the end of the day—before going to bed— explain how you feel about this routine:
  - Exercising early in the morning–Hot water– Breakfast,
  - Hot water–Lunch (4 hours later),
  - Hot water–Healthy snack (4 hours later),
  - Hot water–Dinner (3 hours later).

- How are your energy levels when you're through? How about your motivation levels?

- Do you feel good about yourself? On a scale of 0 to 10 (0 being bad and 10 being fabulous), how would you rank your mood right now?

7-Day Weight Loss Challenge

<u>DAY 5</u>:

Run to Your Health and Heart

Cardio Time

On Day 4 you got a general list of exercises to work with, and on Day 5 you're just going to be adding to that list. But this time, it's an exercise with an immediate benefit: a **healthy heart**. Yes, we're talking about cardio.

One of the easiest, and definitely most accessible, cardio exercises you can do is running. You don't even have to be like preparing for a marathon—you run for 30, 20, or even 15 minutes and still get results. And you can do it anywhere—if you're nervous about running outside by yourself, you can go to the gym and use a good old treadmill or even run in place in your own living room.

Running is a good middle or end-of-the-week exercise because it helps you lower your stress levels and will help keep you from becoming overwhelmed before you reach the finish line. A 2013 study in Medicine & Science in Sports & Exercise, using rats and mice as test subjects, discovered that running on a wheel actually generated effects similar to those produced by anti-depressants. As a result of the study, the researchers concluded that physical activity was an effective treatment for issues like stress and depression that contribute to weight gain from overeating as a way of coping.

To incorporate these effects into your own program, it's best to start slowly, with a 10 to 15-minute session. The ideal way to do this is to start either on an in-home or gym treadmill or by running in place right in your own living room.

But let's face it: running in place can be, well, boring. To make things a little more interesting, then, try timing your run with a music soundtrack. Depending on the length of your run (again, a 10-15 minute session is good to start with) and the songs, set yourself up a 3-4 song track to listen to while you run—not only will it give you a rhythm and a timer but it'll also help you forget about the strain on your legs, your joints, and your lungs.

10 or 15 minutes may not seem like much (or too much for the slobs), but, by making running a part of your weekly routine, you can gradually get your body (especially your heart) used to the activity and the strain. The trick to this is to add 5 minutes (remember, baby steps) each time you feel ready to go a little farther. Keep this up and it won't be long before you're fit to run a marathon!

Exercise: Run! Run! Run!

Try to content yourself by adding the following routine to your plan:

Run in place for 10 minutes. Pick some rhythmic music—such as techno music, for instance (make sure it will last 10 minutes).

- Did 10 minutes of running make you sweat? If so, was it a little or a lot?

- Put your hand on your chest. Is your heart rate higher than usual?

- Did you end the session with a smile, or did you stumble weakly to your fridge for water?

- Describe how you feel as you carry on with your day. Do you feel more active after your exercise? More motivated? Explain.

7-Day Weight Loss Challenge

DAY 6:

Combine End of the Week Relaxation with Workout

The One All-in-One Body Workout

If you had to choose <u>one exercise</u> to look healthy, feel healthy, be healthy - pick **Pilates**. *Out of all the exercises out there, why Pilates?*

Pilates is an exercise very similar to yoga, the only difference being that it promotes the abdomen, obliques, lower back, inner and outer thighs, glutes, etc. In other words, it focuses on your body core. Named after its inventor, Joseph Pilates (a carpenter turned gymnast), it was designed for injured dancers, and many of the moves were, in fact, inspired by yoga or patterned after the movements of animals such as swans, seals, and big cats.

The reason we've put emphasis on Pilates is that it's the perfect type of exercise for body definition, and, unlike standard toning, it also helps correct posture, a double whammy.

As Jillian Hessel, a Los Angeles-based Pilates teacher with 26 years' experience, says, "Pilates can help build and maintain lean muscle mass while you are losing weight, help to realign posture as the body's center of gravity changes, promote long, elegant posture and graceful, flowing movement, and keep you centered and energized—all at the same time."

To get the best results, schedule your Pilates session for the end of the week—Day 5 is perfect for most people, since they're done with work and can focus on a slower, more relaxing type of exercise. (*Note: During Week 1 you'll be doing Pilates on Day 6, but since you won't have to repeat the procedure for Day 1 next week, Pilates will land on Day 5 instead.) Also, even though Pilates doesn't directly emphasize any kind of spiritual wellness, its "breathing-through exercise" and smooth, flowing movements can give you a sense of tranquility and concentration you can't get from your Monday aerobics session.

A Pilates session should normally last up to 1 hour. In the end, you'll have better flexibility and better posture—which is always a help when losing weight and trying to adjust yourself to a new body. It's not even a harsh or strenuous workout, yet Joseph Pilates himself stated that his technique could give you noticeable results in just 30 sessions. Taken all in all, if you want to combine burning calories with building leaner muscles, you just can't get much better than Pilates.

If you're ready to start practicing it on your own, here are some Pilates exercises (each exercise lasts about 5 minutes, more or less):

Pilates Workout 1: The Pelvic Curl

–Lie on your back with your knees bent and your feet flat on the floor. Make sure your feet, ankles, and knees are aligned and a hip-distance apart. This exercise starts in <u>neutral spine</u>. In neutral spine, the natural curves of the spine are present so that the lower back is not pressed into the mat.

–Next, begin <u>sequential breathing</u>. Inhale deeply—through your chest, your stomach, then down to the pelvic bowl. Exhale following the same sequence, releasing the breath from the pelvic bowl, then the stomach, then finally from the chest.

–Inhale again.

–Exhale. After this, start your <u>pelvic tilt</u> by engaging the abdominal muscles and pulling your belly button down toward your spine. Let that action continue so the abs press the lower spine into the floor. In the pelvic tilt position, your back is very long against the floor and the pelvis is tilted so that the pubic bone is a little higher than the hip bones.

–Inhale.

–Press down through your feet, allowing the tailbone to begin curling up toward the ceiling. The hips raise, then the lower spine, then, finally, the middle spine. Make sure to keep your legs parallel throughout the entire exercise.

–You'll come to rest on your shoulder blades, with a nice straight line from your hips to your shoulders—do not arch beyond this point. Be sure to support this movement with the abdominals and hamstrings.

–Exhale.

–As you let your breath go, use abdominal control to roll the spine back down to the floor.

–Begin with the upper back and work your way down, vertebrae by vertebrae, until the lower spine settles to the floor.

–Inhale.

–Release to neutral spine. Prepare to repeat the exercise by initiating the pelvic tilt on the exhale.

(Repeat this exercise 3 to 5 times).

Pilates Workout 2: The Hundred

–Lie on your back with your legs bent in <u>tabletop position</u> (legs raised and bent at the knees so that the shins and ankles are parallel to the floor).

–Inhale.

–Exhale. Bring your head up—making sure to keep your chin down—and, using your abdominal muscles, curl your upper spine up off the floor to the base of your shoulder blades. Keep the shoulders sliding down and engaged in the back. Your eyes should be pointed down into the scoop of the abs.

–Inhale, staying in the previous position.

–Exhale. At the same time, deepen the pull of the abs and extend your arms and legs. Your legs reach toward the point where the wall and ceiling meet in front of you. You can adjust them if need be, either higher for a bit of a break or lower for more advanced work.

–Your legs should be as low as you can hold them without shaking and without causing the lower spine to pull up off the mat.

–Your arms extend straight and low, just a few inches off floor, fingertips reaching for the far wall.

–Hold your position.

–Take 5 short breaths in and 5 short breaths out. At the same time, move your arms in a controlled up and down motion.

–Keep your shoulders and neck relaxed—your abdominal muscles should be doing all the work.

–Do a cycle of 10 full breaths. Each cycle is a sequence of in-out breaths.

–The arms pump up and down—about a 6-8 inch pump— synchronized with your breathing.

–Keep your abs scooped and your back flat on the floor. Your head here is an extension of your spine, with the gaze (eyes) down.

Breathing big is important—make sure you breathe into your back and sides.

–To finish: Keep your spine curved as you bring your knees in toward your chest. Grasp your knees and roll your upper spine and head down to the floor. Take a deep breath—in and out.

Pilates Workout 3: The Single-leg Stretch

–To prepare for this exercise, lie on your back with your legs in the tabletop position.

–Take a few moments to breathe deeply—as if you're trying to get air to the back and lower abs.

–Inhale.

–Exhale. Pull your abs in—taking your belly button down toward your spine—as you curl your head and shoulders up to the tips of the shoulder blades. As you curl up, your left leg extends at a 45-degree angle.

–The right leg remains in tabletop position, the right hand grasping the right ankle and the left hand moving to the right knee.

–You'll maintain your upper-body curve throughout the exercise, but be sure to keep your shoulders relaxed.

–Inhale. Switch legs on a <u>two-part inhale</u>. Bring air in as the left knee comes in, then bring more air in as you gently pulse that knee toward you. Now the left hand moves to the left ankle and the right hand to the left knee.

–Exhale. Switch legs, bringing the right leg in with a two-part exhale-pulse and stretching out the left leg.

–The hand-to-leg coordination continues with the hand corresponding to the bent leg going to the ankle and the other hand moving to the inside of the knee.

–Repeat. Switch legs up to 10 times. Stop the exercise if you're feeling tension in your shoulders and neck, or if your lower back is taking the strain.

Pilates Workout 4: The Spine Stretch

–Inhale, extending your arms out in front of you at shoulder height.

–As a modification here, you can place your fingertips on the floor in front of you (between your legs).

–Exhale as you lengthen (stretch) your spine to curve forward.

–Now, release your hips as you keep your shoulders down and reach your fingers toward your toes.

–Inhale, and try to reach further (don't strain yourself, though) as you enjoy the fullness of your stretch.

–Exhale, initiating your return by using the lower abdominals to bring the pelvis upright, then roll up through the spine to a sitting position.

Pilates Workout 5: Swimming Exercises

–Lie on your stomach with your legs straight and together.

–Keep your shoulder blades settled in your back—shoulders well away from your ears—then stretch your arms straight overhead.

–Pull your abs in, lifting your belly button up and away from the floor.

–Reaching out from center, extend your arms and legs so far in opposite directions that they come naturally up off the floor. At the same time, get so much length in your spine (elongate it) that your head moves up off the mat as an extension of your backbone. Keep your face down toward the mat, but make sure not to crease your neck (to prevent injury).

–Continue to stretch your arms and legs out from your center, at the same time alternating right arm/left leg, then left arm/right leg, pulling them up and down in small pulses.

(Do 2 or 3 cycles of this.)

Pilates Workout 6: Plank Exercise

–Get on your knees and walk your hands out along the floor, allowing your legs to stretch out behind you. Place your forearms parallel to each other on the floor. (Making a fist with the hands can be helpful here.) Make sure your shoulders are directly over your elbows.

–Lift your belly up as you extend your spine. Make sure to keep the pressure out of your lower back by pulling up with your lower abs.

–Position your pubic bone to the floor and allow your tailbone to move down toward the floor as well.

–Broaden your shoulder blades and collarbone, making sure your shoulders are away from your ears.

–Hold the pose for 30 seconds, remembering to breathe fully.

–As soon as you feel your weight starting to drop into your shoulders and arms, release, rest, then try the position once more.

Pilates Workout 7: The Saw Exercise

–Sit up straight.

–Your legs should be extended in front of you, about a shoulder-width apart.

–Stretch your arms out to the sides, making sure they're even with your shoulders.

–Inhale. Stretch yourself up taller as you turn your whole torso, using your abs to keep your hips even with each other.

–Exhale. Let your gaze (your eyes) follow your back hand (the hand that's pointing behind you at this stage) as you turn, spiraling your upper torso so you're almost curling into yourself.

–Allow the stretch to take you forward as you reach the little finger of your front hand across the outside of the opposite foot.

–Exhale once more, and try to reach a little further this time.

Exercise: Practice Pilates

Take one hour to practice the Pilates exercises named above, then answer the following questions:

- How relaxed are you after the practice? (Rank your mood from 0 to 10. 0 being tense and 10 being totally relaxed.)

- Do your muscles feel more stimulated now? Explain.

- Can you notice any improvement in posture—even though this is just the first session? Explain.

7-Day Weight Loss Challenge

DAY 7:

Reflexive Actions

Habits to Incorporate

After six days of sweat, hot water, and good work, you've finally reached Day 7. Since today is reserved for rest, however, we're going to leave exercises for today and introduce you to a few more habits that will be useful during your program. Remember, you've been very active this week, but that's no excuse for letting yourself go now.

Read this list through, then, and try to incorporate the suggestions as part of your daily life:

–**Keep your stomach tucked in**, at all times. Keeping your core taut can only help your stomach muscles tighten and maybe even lose a few inches. One way to achieve this is to breathe slowly in and out, sucking your stomach in on the in-breath—smoothly, though; you don't want to force it. Remember, this should eventually become a reflex—you don't want to start out by injuring yourself.

–**Keep yourself well hydrated**. The hot water you've added to your routine probably isn't enough for your body to survive on, so drinking cool or room temperature water is still important. Plus, there's nothing appealing about hot water after a warm and sweaty workout, is there? And practically no other liquid works as well as water to hydrate you—especially try to avoid those with sugar, artificial flavors, and caffeine.

–**Avoid eating immediately before working out.** Having a full stomach really makes exercising hard, making you feel incredibly heavy and sometimes even nauseous. If you have to eat in the morning before exercising, make sure you allow 3 to 4 hours for digestion before you start your workout.

–**Chew your food slowly.** Eating fast can only put so much strain on your stomach, and besides, eating slowly allows you to enjoy your food more fully and might even encourage you to eat smaller quantities.

–**Don't use the scale all the time.** The only time you should use it is in the morning, when your stomach is empty. This is the only time your real weight will be measured.

–**Cook your own meals.** This way you can personally control how much grease, salt, or sugar is added to your food.

–**Getting to bed early and waking up early** helps you regenerate better and helps your body store enough strength for the day to come.

These habits should become an everyday part of life for you from now on—even on the days when you don't have to exercise.

So, for Day 7, drink your usual 4 to 6 glasses of hot water, eat 4 times a day (respecting the 4-hour gap between meals, just like any other day), and work on respecting these new guidelines.

The Final Steps: In the Weeks to Come

Week 1 was your weight-loss package. In other words, these new habits, exercises, and eating changes are the tools you've received, with different combinations and options for you to choose from every week until you reach your goal.

That said, here are three important things to remember when you organize next week's program:

1.) Keep your 4-6 glasses of hot water part of your daily routine, and follow the suggestions listed on Day 7 (cook your own meals, get to sleep early, don't use the scale all the time, etc.).

2.) This week you've learned to substitute your meals, replacing ones rich in carbs and sugar with healthier alternatives. In the weeks to come, this substitution has to become an automatic, unconscious reaction (meaning that you shouldn't have to think twice about choosing between a doughnut or a cup of yogurt—the immediate choice should be the yogurt).

3.) When it comes to exercise, do your best to organize your sessions according to the plan listed below. Remember, you don't have to repeat the steps for Day 1 next week (of mentally prepping yourself since you've already done so for this first week of the seven days), so you'll have an extra day to work with. Given that, your workout schedule for the following weeks should look something like this:

Monday: Start up your day with some motivation

–7:00: Wake up.

–7:10: Start your 30 to 40 minute aerobics session.

–8:00: Drink some water to cool off, then have your glass of hot water (flavored with a slice of lemon) to get your metabolism going. Have your healthy breakfast for the day.

Tuesday: Relax your senses and stretch your body

–7:00: Wake up.

–7:10: Have a 50-60 minute yoga session.

–8:10: Drink your metabolism-boosting mixture, then eat breakfast.

Wednesday: Release tension with weight training

–7:00: Wake up.

–7:10: Begin your 20 to 30 minute weight session (you're not a body builder—don't overdo it).

–7:40: Hydrate yourself with a glass of water. 5 minutes later, have your glass of hot water, then eat breakfast.

Thursday: Building lean muscle and relaxation . . . all at the same time

–7:00: Wake up.

−7: 10: Begin your 1-hour Pilates session.

−8:10: Have your hot glass of water, then eat a healthy, natural breakfast.

Friday: End your week with some cardio

−7:00: Wake up.

−7:10: Begin your cardio session. Remember, with running you can start small at first, adding additional minutes each week. So, if you started at 10 minutes during the first week, you can add 5 more minutes this week, and so on until you find a timing you consider fair enough (it could be 20 minutes, 30 minutes, or more, depending on what you prefer).

−Boost your metabolism like you did during the previous days, then eat your breakfast. Don't forget to hydrate yourself immediately after the session.

This type of scheduling shows you how to alternate from rough, demanding workouts (like aerobics, weight lifting, etc.) to smoother, slower, and more relaxing ones (such as Pilates and yoga). It makes a good strategy as it not only allows you to benefit from different disciplines, at the same time enhancing your mind and body, but also allows you to help your body recuperate between sessions.

- For example, if you start with aerobics on Monday, your Tuesday Pilates session will help you stretch your body and joints and breathe better so you can carry on the next day (Wednesday) "rejuvenated" and ready for your more difficult routines.

Make sure you carry on with the same diet and workout routine till the first results show up (3 months later or however long you've planned). Later you may need to switch up your exercise a little, since eventually you're not pushing yourself any more, but you haven't reached that point yet.

Remember, weight-loss demands patience, and sticking to one solid routine will make it that much easier to live with. Also, when you reach the third month of the program, recalculate your BMI to check your current weight status.

You are now done with your 7-day program. Nothing is monotonous with a weight-loss program, as one routine will lead you to different, but satisfactory results each week.

Nothing should be seen as a challenge at this point—unless you want it to be one, of course. Learn to enjoy every single day of your program.

7-Day Weight Loss Challenge

Challenge Complete:

Weight Reduced

You've completed your first 7-day weight-loss challenge, but remember, weight loss is not an overnight thing—it takes time. Losing weight shouldn't be something you expect to achieve, then immediately switch back to your old habits. It should be adapted into your lifestyle, as natural a part of is as brushing your teeth every morning and night. So, when you finish this first week, keep challenging yourself to keep up your program, making every 7 days a new personal achievement.

Don't forget, though, that this 7-day challenge is by no means set in stone. Change things up if you have to. Alternate your exercises, and above all, **make sure your diet suits you**. If you get bored eating the same things over and over again, experiment with new healthy foods or new dishes. This week is about *discovery*. Discover what you need and works for you.

Sure, sometimes researching and setting up a program can be stressful. There's so much different advice out there, and information seems to become obsolete really fast—often, when it comes to weight loss, what was the norm 10 years ago is invalidated today.

You can make it easier on yourself, however, if you keep in mind that there will always be three things your body needs, no matter what. These three things are 1.) water, 2.) nutrients from healthy, natural foods, and 3.) exercise.

People tend to blame weight problems on the quality of the food we eat, but our sedentary lifestyle also plays a huge role. Think about it: in the past, people were much more active and ate organic, and often unprepared, foods; today on the other hand, we have desk jobs, video games, and TVs, and we're content to eat synthetic foods made from ingredients most people can't even pronounce.

In other words, weight problems are essentially a product of our modern lifestyle. If we want to be healthy, we need to readopt the good old ways—ways that let people enjoy the things that really matter, such as health and discovering new things.

So, stick to your resolve and follow your personalized weight-loss program to discover a healthier, happier life that will bring you closer to the natural ways we used to enjoy. Good luck!

<u>Your Feedback:</u>

Was Your Challenge Accomplished?

Congratulations on completing all your challenges! You should be proud of yourself for making it this far. For that, give yourself a big pat on the back! :)

Now, we have a huge favor that we would like to ask you. We want to know: have you accomplished the goal you established when you began this trial?

No two people are the same, so results will always vary.

If you have seen the results you wanted, give yourself another pat on the back, and please kindly share your testimonial wherever you purchased this book. If you let us know about it, we have a small free gift to offer you as a token of our appreciation.

However, if you aren't satisfied in any way, we urge you to please contact us directly to let us know what could have been different to help you achieve better results. We want to know if there is any way we can further help you.

Plus we are very easy to get a hold of online!

Official Website:
http://www.ChallengeSelf.com

Social Media:
https://www.facebook.com/ChallengeSelf
https://twitter.com/MyChallengeSelf
https://plus.google.com/+Challengeself

"YOU" are our main priority, and we're all here for you!

Take care! And always challenge yourself!